PLANT BASED
INSULIN RESISTANCE DIET
FOR PCOS

Vegan Recipes to Prevent Prediabetes, Manage Weight, and Boost Fertility

LAKEISHA OWENS

TABLE OF CONTENT

INTRODUCTION

PCOS is a multifaceted condition with a spectrum of symptoms that can affect women of reproductive age, leading to challenges such as irregular menstrual cycles, infertility, weight gain, acne, and hirsutism. At the heart of many PCOS cases is insulin resistance, a condition where the body's cells don't respond effectively to insulin, leading to elevated blood sugar levels and a host of metabolic issues. Research has shown that diet plays a crucial role in managing insulin sensitivity and can be a powerful tool in controlling PCOS symptoms.

This book is grounded in the latest scientific research and combines the principles of vegan nutrition with strategies to combat insulin resistance. We delve into the benefits of a vegan diet, not only for PCOS and insulin resistance but also for overall health, including weight management, cardiovascular health, and environmental sustainability.

Our focus on a plant-based diet for managing PCOS is deliberate and informed. A vegan diet, rich in whole foods, provides an abundance of fiber, vitamins, minerals, and phytonutrients that can help regulate blood sugar levels, support hormonal balance, and reduce inflammation.

However, adopting a vegan diet, especially for managing a condition like PCOS, comes with its challenges. Ensuring adequate intake of essential nutrients, balancing macronutrients, and choosing foods that naturally support insulin sensitivity are pivotal aspects that this book addresses comprehensively.

Our goal is to empower you with the recipes you need to take control of your PCOS symptoms through a healthy, sustainable vegan diet. Whether you are newly diagnosed with PCOS, struggling with insulin resistance, or a long-term vegan looking to optimize your diet for PCOS management, this book is for you.

Embark on this journey with us to transform your health, one plant-based meal at a time. Together, we will navigate the path to a healthier, happier you.

HAPPY COOKING

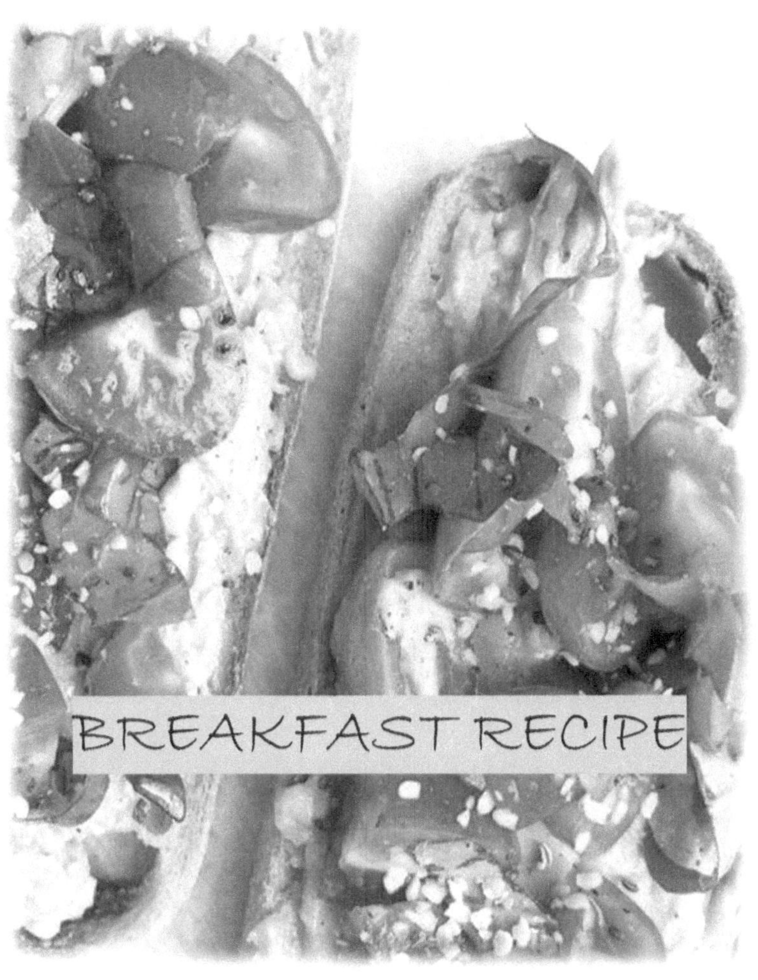

BREAKFAST RECIPE

BREAKFAST RECIPE
Chia and Flaxseed Pudding

Ingredients:

2 tablespoons chia seeds

1 tablespoon ground flaxseeds

1 cup unsweetened almond milk

½ teaspoon vanilla extract

Stevia or monk fruit to taste

Mixed berries for topping

Instructions:

In a bowl, mix the chia seeds, ground flaxseeds, almond milk, and vanilla extract.

Sweeten with stevia or monk fruit according to taste.

Give everything a good stir, then refrigerate for at least two hours or overnight.

Serve with a topping of mixed berries.

Tofu Scramble with Spinach

Ingredients:

200g firm tofu, crumbled.

1 tablespoon olive oil

½ teaspoon turmeric

½ teaspoon garlic powder

1 cup spinach, fresh

Salt and pepper to taste

Avocado slices for serving.

Instructions:

Heat the olive oil in a pan over moderate heat.

Add the crumbled tofu, turmeric, and garlic powder.

Cook for 5-7 minutes, stirring frequently.

Add the spinach and cook until wilted.

Season with salt and pepper.

Serve with avocado slices on the side.

Low-Carb Coconut Flour Pancakes

Ingredients:

½ cup coconut flour

1 teaspoon baking powder

2 flax eggs (2 tablespoons ground flaxseed mixed with 6 tablespoons water, let sit for 5 minutes)

¾ cup unsweetened almond milk

1 tablespoon coconut oil, melted.

1 teaspoon vanilla extract

Stevia or monk fruit to taste

Instructions:

Combine the baking powder and coconut flour in a bowl.

Add the flax eggs, almond milk, melted coconut oil, and vanilla extract.

Mix until smooth.

Heat a non-stick pan over medium heat and pour batter to form pancakes.

Simmer until bubbles appear, then turn and continue cooking until golden.

Serve with sugar-free vegan syrup or fresh berries.

Avocado and Tomato Toast

Ingredients:

2 slices of whole grain, low-GI bread

1 ripe avocado

1 tomato, sliced.

Salt, pepper, and chili flakes to taste

A squeeze of lemon juice

Instructions:

Toast the bread slices until golden.

Spread the avocado on the toasted bread after mashing it.

Top with tomato slices, and season with salt, pepper, and chili flakes.

Finally, drizzle a little lemon juice on top.

Berry Smoothie with Spinach

Ingredients:

1 cup mixed berries (strawberries, blueberries, raspberries)

1 cup spinach

1 tablespoon chia seeds

1 cup unsweetened almond milk

Stevia or monk fruit to taste

Instructions:

Blend all ingredients until smooth.

Add ice for a colder smoothie if desired.

Sweeten with stevia or monk fruit to taste.

Almond Butter and Banana Oatmeal

Ingredients:

½ cup rolled oats

1 cup unsweetened almond milk

1 tablespoon almond butter

1 banana, sliced.

Cinnamon to taste

Instructions:

Cook the oats in almond milk according to package instructions.

Stir in the almond butter and top with banana slices.

Sprinkle cinnamon on top before serving.

Savory Mushroom and Kale Breakfast Bowl

Ingredients:

1 cup kale, chopped.

1 cup mushrooms, sliced.

1 tablespoon olive oil

2 tablespoons nutritional yeast

Salt and pepper to taste

½ avocado, sliced

Instructions:

Heat the olive oil in a pan over moderate heat.

When the mushrooms begin to soften, add them and simmer.

When the kale has wilted, add it and simmer.

Add the nutritional yeast, pepper, and salt and stir.

Serve in a bowl topped with avocado slices.

Zucchini and Carrot Fritters

Ingredients:

1 zucchini, grated.

1 carrot, grated.

2 tablespoons ground flaxseed mixed with 6 tablespoons water (flax egg)

¼ cup chickpea flour

Salt and pepper to taste

1 tablespoon olive oil for cooking

Instructions:

Squeeze the excess moisture from the grated zucchini and carrot.

Mix the zucchini, carrot, flax egg, chickpea flour, salt, and pepper in a bowl.

Form into patties.

Heat olive oil in a pan over moderate heat. Cook the fritters until golden on both sides.

Vegan Yogurt with Nuts and Seeds

Ingredients:

1 cup unsweetened vegan yogurt (coconut, almond, or soy)

1 tablespoon pumpkin seeds

1 tablespoon sunflower seeds

1 tablespoon almonds, chopped.

A pinch of cinnamon

Instructions:

In a bowl, combine the vegan yogurt with the seeds and chopped almonds.

Sprinkle cinnamon on top.

Stir gently before eating.

Sweet Potato and Black Bean Breakfast Burritos

Ingredients:

1 medium sweet potato cubed and roasted.

½ cup black beans, cooked

2 whole grain or low-carb vegan tortillas

¼ cup avocado, mashed

1 teaspoon cumin

Salt and pepper to taste

Fresh cilantro for garnish

Instructions:

Mix the roasted sweet potato cubes with black beans, cumin, salt, and pepper.

Warm the tortillas slightly, then spread each with mashed avocado.

Divide the sweet potato and black bean mixture between the tortillas, roll them up.

Garnish with fresh cilantro before serving.

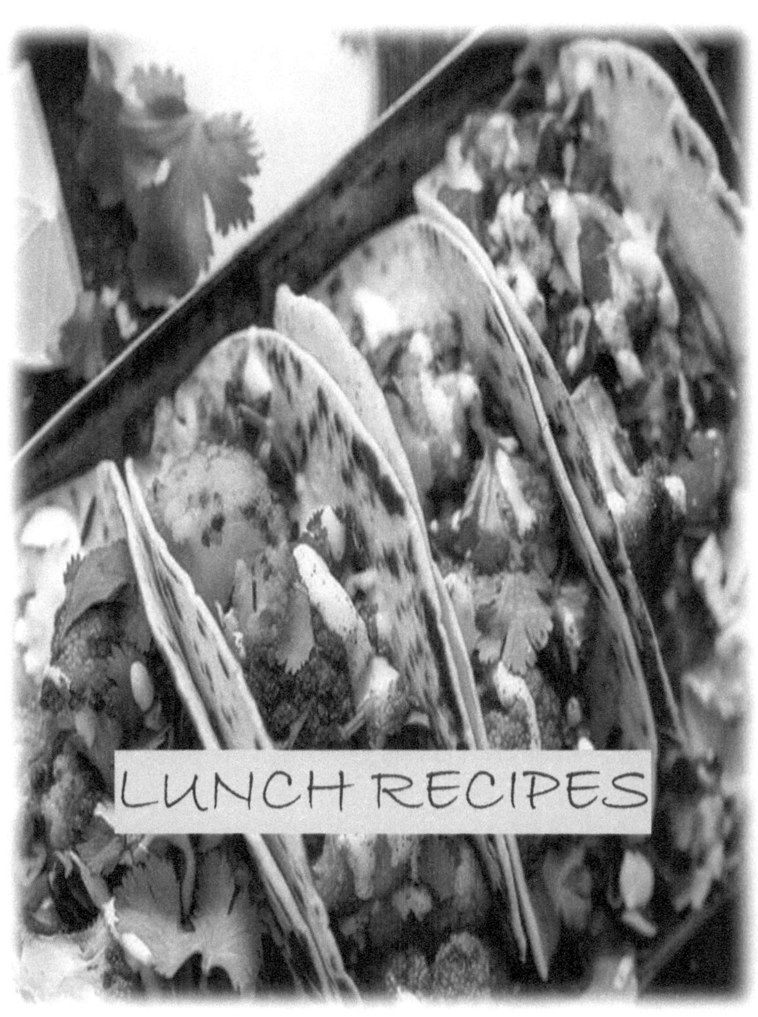
LUNCH RECIPES

LUNCH RECIPES

Lentil and Vegetable Stew

Ingredients:

1 cup dried lentils, rinsed.

1 onion, diced.

2 carrots, diced.

2 celery stalks, diced.

3 garlic cloves, minced.

1 can diced tomatoes (no added salt)

4 cups vegetable broth

1 teaspoon cumin

1 teaspoon paprika

Salt and pepper to taste

2 tablespoons olive oil

Fresh parsley for garnish

Instructions:

Heat olive oil in a large pot over moderate heat.

Add onion, carrots, celery, and garlic.

Cook until vegetables are soft.

Add lentils, diced tomatoes, vegetable broth, cumin, and paprika. Stir well.

Bring to a boil, then reduce heat and simmer covered for 25-30 minutes, until lentils are tender.

Season with salt and pepper.

Garnish with fresh parsley before serving.

Chickpea Salad Sandwich

Ingredients:

1 can chickpeas drained and rinsed.

1/4 cup vegan mayonnaise

1 tablespoon Dijon mustard

1 celery stalk, diced.

1/4 red onion finely chopped.

Salt and pepper to taste

Whole grain bread

Lettuce leaves and tomato slices for serving.

Instructions:

Using a potato masher or fork, mash the chickpeas in a bowl. Mix in vegan mayonnaise, Dijon mustard, celery, red onion, salt, and pepper until well combined.

Serve the chickpea salad on whole grain bread with lettuce and tomato slices.

Stuffed Bell Peppers

Ingredients:

4 bell peppers, tops cut off and seeds removed.

1 cup brown rice, cooked.

1 can black beans drained and rinsed.

1 cup corn kernels

1 cup salsa

1 teaspoon chili powder

1 teaspoon cumin

Salt and pepper to taste

Fresh cilantro for garnish

Instructions:

Preheat oven to 375°F (190°C).

In a bowl, mix the cooked brown rice, black beans, corn, salsa, chili powder, cumin, salt, and pepper.

After stuffing the bell peppers with the mixture, put them in a baking tray.

Cover with foil and bake for 30-35 minutes, until peppers are tender.

Garnish with fresh cilantro before serving.

Vegan Cauliflower Tacos

Ingredients:

1 head cauliflower, cut into small florets.

2 tablespoons olive oil

1 teaspoon chili powder

1 teaspoon paprika

1/2 teaspoon garlic powder

Salt and pepper to taste

Corn tortillas

Avocado slices, lime wedges, and fresh cilantro for serving.

Instructions:

Preheat oven to 400°F (200°C).

Toss the cauliflower florets with olive oil, chili powder, paprika, garlic powder, salt, and pepper.

Spread on a baking sheet and roast for 25-30 minutes, until tender and slightly caramelized.

Serve the roasted cauliflower in corn tortillas, topped with avocado slices, a squeeze of lime, and fresh cilantro.

Spinach and Mushroom Pasta

Ingredients:

8 ounces whole grain pasta

2 tablespoons olive oil

2 garlic cloves, minced.

2 cups mushrooms, sliced.

4 cups spinach leaves

Salt and pepper to taste

Nutritional yeast for serving.

Instructions:

Pasta should be cooked as directed on the package; drain and set aside.

In the same pot, heat olive oil over moderate heat.

Add garlic and mushrooms; cook until mushrooms are soft.

Add spinach and cook until wilted. Season with salt and pepper.

Mix the cooked pasta with the mixture of spinach and mushrooms.

Serve sprinkled with nutritional yeast.

Vegan Buddha Bowl

Ingredients:

1 cup kale, chopped.

1 small, sweet potato cubed and roasted.

1/2 cup chickpeas, roasted.

1/2 avocado, sliced.

1/2 cup cucumber, sliced.

1/4 cup red cabbage, shredded.

2 tablespoons hummus

Lemon wedge for serving.

Salt, pepper, and olive oil

Instructions:

Place kale at the bottom of a bowl and drizzle with olive oil, salt, and pepper.

Arrange the roasted sweet potato, roasted chickpeas, avocado slices, cucumber slices, and shredded red cabbage on top of the kale.

Dollop hummus on top.

Serve with a lemon wedge on the side.

Vegan Lentil Soup

Ingredients:

1 cup red lentils, rinsed.

1 onion, diced.

2 carrots, diced.

2 celery stalks, diced.

3 garlic cloves, minced.

4 cups vegetable broth

1 can diced tomatoes (no added salt)

1 teaspoon cumin

1 teaspoon coriander

Salt and pepper to taste

2 tablespoons olive oil

Lemon wedges for serving.

Instructions:

Heat olive oil in a large pot over moderate heat.

Add onion, carrots, celery, and garlic; cook until softened.

Add lentils, vegetable broth, diced tomatoes, cumin, and coriander. Bring to a boil, then simmer for 20-25 minutes, until lentils are tender.

Season with salt and pepper.

Serve with a lemon wedge.

Avocado and Bean Wrap

Ingredients:

Whole grain wraps

1 avocado, mashed.

1/2 cup black beans drained and rinsed.

1/4 cup corn kernels

1/2 tomato, diced.

Lettuce leaves

Salt and pepper to taste

Instructions:

Spread mashed avocado on a whole grain wrap.

Top with black beans, corn, diced tomato, and lettuce.

Season with salt and pepper.

Roll up the wrap tightly and serve.

Eggplant and Chickpea Curry

Ingredients:

1 large eggplant, cubed.
1 can chickpeas drained and rinsed.
1 onion, diced.
2 garlic cloves, minced.
1 can coconut milk
2 tablespoons curry powder
1 teaspoon turmeric
Salt and pepper to taste
2 tablespoons olive oil
Fresh cilantro for garnish

Instructions:

In a big pan, warm up the olive oil over medium heat.

Add the garlic and onion and sauté until tender.

When the eggplant begins to soften, add it and simmer.

Stir in chickpeas, coconut milk, curry powder, and turmeric. Season with salt and pepper.

Bring to a simmer and cook for 20-25 minutes, until the eggplant is tender, and the flavors are well blended.

Garnish with fresh cilantro before serving.

This curry pairs wonderfully with a side of brown rice or a whole grain flatbread to soak up the delicious sauce.

Zucchini Noodle Stir-Fry

Ingredients:

2 large zucchinis, spiralized

1 bell pepper thinly sliced.

1 carrot, julienned.

1/2 onion thinly sliced.

2 garlic cloves, minced.

1 tablespoon ginger, minced.

1/4 cup soy sauce (low sodium)

1 tablespoon sesame oil

1 tablespoon olive oil

Sesame seeds for garnish

Instructions:

Heat olive oil in a large skillet over moderate heat.
Add onion, garlic, and ginger, sauté until fragrant.
Add bell pepper and carrot; cook until slightly softened.
Spiralize the zucchini noodles and turn the heat up to medium-high.

Stir-fry for 2-3 minutes, until just tender.

Drizzle with soy sauce and sesame oil, tossing everything together to coat well.

After cooking for one more minute, turn off the heat.

Serve the stir-fry garnished with sesame seeds.

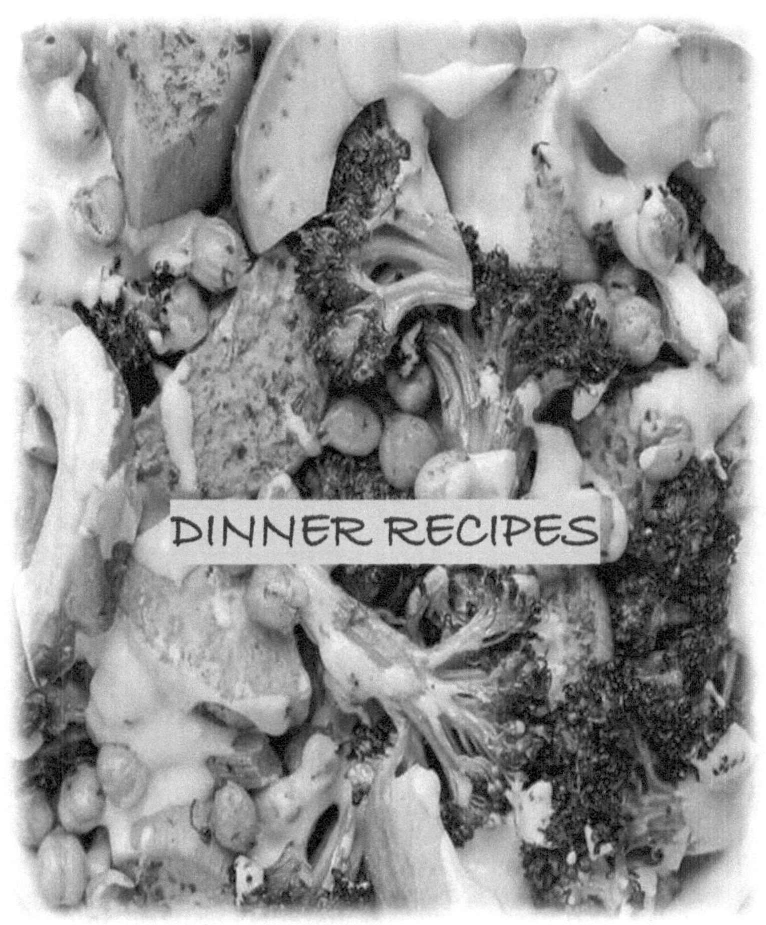
DINNER RECIPES

DINNER RECIPES

Tofu Stir-Fry with Broccoli and Bell Peppers

Ingredients:

1 block firm tofu pressed and cubed.

2 cups broccoli florets

1 red bell pepper, sliced.

1 yellow bell pepper, sliced.

2 tablespoons soy sauce (low sodium)

1 tablespoon sesame oil

1 tablespoon olive oil

2 garlic cloves, minced.

1 teaspoon grated ginger

Sesame seeds for garnish

Instructions:

Heat olive oil in a large skillet over medium-high heat.

Stir-fry the tofu cubes until they turn golden brown.

Remove from the skillet and set aside.

Add ginger, garlic, and sesame oil to the same skillet.

Sauté until aromatic, about 1 minute.

Add broccoli and bell peppers.

Stir-fry for about 5 minutes, until vegetables are tender but still crisp.

Return the tofu to the skillet, add soy sauce, and toss everything together.

Cook for another 2-3 minutes.

Garnish with sesame seeds before serving.

Vegan Lentil Bolognese

Ingredients:

1 cup red lentils, rinsed.

1 onion, diced.
2 garlic cloves, minced.
1 carrot, diced.
1 celery stalk, diced.
1 can diced tomatoes.
2 tablespoons tomato paste
1 teaspoon dried oregano
1 teaspoon dried basil
Salt and pepper to taste
2 tablespoons olive oil
Whole wheat spaghetti

Instructions:

Heat olive oil in a large pan over moderate heat.

Add onion, garlic, carrot, and celery, and sauté until softened.

Stir in lentils, diced tomatoes, tomato paste, oregano, basil, salt, and pepper.

Add water if necessary to cover the lentils.

Bring to a boil, then reduce heat and simmer for 25-30 minutes, until lentils are tender, and sauce has thickened.

Serve over cooked whole wheat spaghetti.

Eggplant Parmesan

Ingredients:

2 large eggplants, sliced into 1/2-inch rounds.
Salt
2 cups marinara sauce
2 cups vegan mozzarella cheese, shredded.
1/2 cup vegan parmesan cheese, grated.
1/2 cup breadcrumbs
2 tablespoons olive oil
Fresh basil for garnish

Instructions:

Preheat oven to 375°F (190°C). Arrange the slices of eggplant on a paper towel and lightly dust with salt. Let sit for 10-15 minutes to draw out moisture, then pat dry.

Arrange eggplant slices in a single layer on a baking sheet. Drizzle with olive oil and bake for 20 minutes, until tender.

Cover the bottom of a baking dish with marinara sauce. Add a layer of baked eggplant slices, then sprinkle with vegan mozzarella and parmesan cheese. Repeat layers until all ingredients are used, finishing with a cheese layer.

Top with breadcrumbs and bake for 25-30 minutes, until golden and bubbly.

Garnish with fresh basil before serving.

Stuffed Acorn Squash

Ingredients:

2 acorn squash halved, and seeds removed.

1 cup wild rice, cooked.

1/2 cup cranberries

1/2 cup pecans, chopped.

1 onion, diced.

2 garlic cloves, minced.

1 apple, diced.

1 teaspoon cinnamon

1/2 teaspoon nutmeg

Salt and pepper to taste

2 tablespoons olive oil

Instructions:

Preheat oven to 375°F (190°C).

Place acorn squash halves cut side up on a baking sheet. Add

a drizzle of olive oil and season with pepper and salt.

Bake for about 25-30 minutes, until tender.

Heat the olive oil in a skillet over medium heat while the squash bakes.

Add onion and garlic, and sauté until translucent.

Add diced apple, cranberries, pecans, cinnamon, and nutmeg.

Cook for another 5 minutes.

Stir in cooked wild rice and cook until everything is heated through.

Season with salt and pepper to taste.

Stuff the baked acorn squash halves with the rice mixture and serve.

Vegan Mushroom Stroganoff

Ingredients:

8 ounces whole wheat pasta

2 tablespoons olive oil

1 onion, diced.

2 garlic cloves, minced.

16 ounces mushrooms, sliced.

1 tablespoon soy sauce (low sodium)

1 teaspoon paprika

1 cup vegetable broth

1/2 cup cashew cream (blend-soaked cashews with water until smooth)

Salt and pepper to taste

Fresh parsley, chopped for garnish.

Instructions:

Pasta should be cooked as directed on the package; drain and set aside.

In a big skillet over medium heat, warm up the olive oil.

Add the garlic and onion and cook until transparent.

When the mushrooms release their moisture and begin to brown, add them and simmer.

Stir in soy sauce and paprika.

Add vegetable broth and bring to a simmer.

Reduce heat and stir in cashew cream.

Cook until the sauce thickens.

Season with salt and pepper.

Toss the pasta with the mushroom sauce.

Garnish with fresh parsley before serving.

Vegan Cauliflower Curry

Ingredients:

1 head cauliflower, cut into florets.

1 can chickpeas drained and rinsed.

1 onion, diced.

2 garlic cloves, minced.

1 can coconut milk

2 tablespoons curry powder

1 teaspoon turmeric

Salt and pepper to taste

2 tablespoons olive oil

Fresh cilantro for garnish

Instructions:

In a big pot, warm up the olive oil over medium heat.

Add the garlic and onion and cook until transparent.

Stir in curry powder and turmeric, cooking for another minute until fragrant.

Add cauliflower, chickpeas, and coconut milk.

Season with salt and pepper.

After bringing to a boil, lower the heat, and simmer the cauliflower for 20 to 25 minutes, or until it becomes soft.

Garnish with fresh cilantro before serving.

This curry is perfectly served over a bed of brown rice or with whole grain naan for a comforting, nutritious meal.

Ingredients:

1 onion, chopped.

2 cloves garlic, minced.

1 bell pepper, chopped.

2 carrots, diced.

2 celery stalks, diced.

1 zucchini, diced.

1 can black beans drained and rinsed.

1 can kidney beans drained and rinsed.

1 can diced tomatoes.

2 tablespoons tomato paste

2 tablespoons chili powder

1 teaspoon cumin

1 teaspoon smoked paprika.

Salt and pepper to taste

2 tablespoons olive oil

Fresh cilantro and avocado for garnish

Instructions:

In a big pot, warm up the olive oil over medium heat.

Add the bell pepper, celery, carrots, onion, and garlic.

Cook until vegetables are softened.

Add zucchini, black beans, kidney beans, diced tomatoes, tomato paste, chili powder, cumin, and smoked paprika.

Season with salt and pepper.

After bringing to a boil, lower the heat, and simmer for 30 minutes while stirring now and then.

Add slices of avocado and fresh cilantro as garnish.

Vegan Sweet Potato Shepherd's Pie

Ingredients:

4 large, sweet potatoes peeled and cubed.

1 onion, diced.

2 cloves garlic, minced.

1 cup frozen mixed vegetables (peas, carrots, corn)

1 can lentils drained and rinsed.

1 tablespoon tomato paste

1 teaspoon thyme

1 teaspoon rosemary

Salt and pepper to taste

2 tablespoons olive oil

1/4 cup almond milk

Instructions:

Preheat oven to 400°F (200°C).

Boil sweet potatoes until tender, then mash with almond milk, salt, and pepper. Set it aside.

Heat olive oil in a pan over medium heat.

Add onion and garlic, and sauté until translucent.

Add mixed vegetables, lentils, tomato paste, thyme, and rosemary.

Cook for 5 minutes, then season with salt and pepper.

Transfer the vegetable mixture to a baking dish.

Top with mashed sweet potatoes, spreading evenly.

Bake for 20 minutes, until the top is slightly golden.

Let it cool for a few minutes before serving.

Vegan Mushroom Fajitas

Ingredients:

2 tablespoons olive oil
3 portobello mushrooms, sliced.
1 red bell pepper, sliced.
1 yellow bell pepper, sliced.
1 onion, sliced.
2 teaspoons chili powder
1 teaspoon cumin
1/2 teaspoon smoked paprika.
Salt and pepper to taste
Whole wheat tortillas
Avocado, lime wedges, and fresh cilantro for serving.

Instructions:

In a large skillet set over medium-high heat, warm the olive oil.

Add mushrooms, bell peppers, and onion. Cook, stirring occasionally, until vegetables are tender and slightly charred.

Stir in chili powder, cumin, smoked paprika, salt, and pepper. Cook for another minute until fragrant.

Serve the vegetable mixture with whole wheat tortillas, topped with avocado slices, a squeeze of lime, and fresh cilantro.

Vegan Eggplant Lasagna

Ingredients:

2 large eggplants sliced lengthwise.
1 cup cashew ricotta (blend-soaked cashews with lemon juice, nutritional yeast, garlic, and salt)
1 jar marinara sauce
2 cups spinach
1 zucchini thinly sliced.
Olive oil for brushing
Salt and pepper to taste
Nutritional yeast for sprinkling

Instructions:

Preheat oven to 375°F (190°C).

Add salt and pepper to the eggplant slices after brushing them with olive oil.

Bake on a baking sheet for 20 minutes, until soft.

Cover the bottom of a baking dish with marinara sauce.

Add a layer of eggplant slices, then spread a layer of cashew ricotta, followed by spinach and zucchini slices.

Repeat layers, finishing with marinara sauce.

Cover with foil and bake for 40 minutes.

Remove foil, sprinkle nutritional yeast on top, and bake for another 10 minutes.

Allow it to cool for a few minutes, then cut into slices and serve.

SOUP RECIPE

SOUP RECIPE

Lentil Vegetable Soup

Ingredients:

1 cup dried lentils, rinsed.

1 onion, chopped.

2 carrots, diced.

2 stalks celery, diced.

2 cloves garlic, minced.

1 can diced tomatoes (no salt added)

6 cups vegetable broth

1 teaspoon cumin

1 teaspoon coriander

2 bay leaves

Salt and pepper to taste

2 cups spinach, chopped.

2 tablespoons olive oil

Instructions:

In a large pot, heat olive oil over moderate heat.

Add onion, carrots, celery, and garlic.

Sauté until vegetables are softened.

Add lentils, diced tomatoes, vegetable broth, cumin, coriander, bay leaves, salt, and pepper.

Bring to a boil.

Reduce heat and simmer, covered, for about 30 minutes or until lentils are tender.

Stir in spinach and cook until wilted.

Remove bay leaves before serving.

Broccoli Almond Soup

Ingredients:

1 tablespoon olive oil

1 onion, chopped.

2 cloves garlic, minced.

4 cups broccoli florets

4 cups vegetable broth

1/2 cup raw almonds, with more to garnish.

Salt and pepper to taste

Almond slices for garnish

Instructions:

Heat olive oil in a large pot over moderate heat.

Add onion and garlic, sauté until translucent.

Add broccoli and vegetable broth.

Bring to a boil, then reduce heat and simmer until broccoli is tender, about 15-20 minutes.

Add almonds to the soup.

Use an immersion blender to puree the soup until smooth.

Season with salt and pepper.

Serve garnished with almond slices.

Spicy Black Bean Soup

Ingredients:

2 cans black beans rinsed and drained.
1 onion, chopped.
2 cloves garlic, minced.
1 bell pepper, chopped.
4 cups vegetable broth
1 teaspoon cumin
1 teaspoon paprika
1/2 teaspoon chili powder (adjust to taste)
Salt and pepper to taste
2 tablespoons olive oil
Fresh cilantro for garnish
Avocado slices for garnish

Instructions:

Heat olive oil in a pot over moderate heat. Add onion, garlic, and bell pepper. Sauté until soft.

Add one can of black beans, vegetable broth, cumin, paprika, chili powder, salt, and pepper.

Bring to a boil, then reduce heat and allow to simmer for 10 minutes.

Using an immersion blender, mix the soup until it is smooth.

Add the remaining can of black beans and heat through.

Serve garnished with fresh cilantro and avocado slices.

Carrot Ginger Soup

Ingredients:

2 tablespoons olive oil

1 onion, chopped.

2 cloves garlic, minced.

6 cups chopped carrots.

4 cups vegetable broth

2 tablespoons grated fresh ginger.

Salt and pepper to taste

Coconut cream for garnish

Instructions:

Heat olive oil in a large pot over moderate heat.

Add onion and garlic, and sauté until translucent.

Add carrots, vegetable broth, and ginger.

Bring to a boil, then simmer until carrots are tender, about 20 minutes.

Blend the soup until smooth using an immersion blender.

Season with salt and pepper.

Serve with a swirl of coconut cream.

Mushroom Barley Soup

Ingredients:

1 cup pearl barley, rinsed.

2 tablespoons olive oil

1 onion, chopped.

2 cloves garlic, minced.

2 cups sliced mushrooms.

6 cups vegetable broth

1 teaspoon thyme

Salt and pepper to taste

Parsley for garnish

Instructions:

In a large pot, heat olive oil over moderate heat.

Add onion, garlic, and mushrooms.

Cook until the mushrooms are soft.

Add barley, vegetable broth, thyme, salt, and pepper. Bring to a boil.

Reduce heat, cover, and simmer for about 40 minutes, or until barley is tender.

Garnish with parsley before serving.

Cauliflower Leek Soup

Ingredients:

1 tablespoon olive oil

1 large leek, cleaned and sliced (white and light green parts only)

2 cloves garlic, minced.

1 head cauliflower, chopped.

5 cups vegetable broth

Salt and pepper to taste

Chives for garnish

Instructions:

Heat olive oil in a large pot over moderate heat.

Add leeks and garlic, sauté until leeks are softened.

Add cauliflower and vegetable broth.

Season with salt and pepper.

Bring to a boil, then simmer until cauliflower is tender, about 20 minutes.

Blend the soup until smooth.

Adjust seasoning as needed.

Garnish with chives before serving.

Sweet Potato and Red Lentil Soup

Ingredients:

1 tablespoon olive oil

1 onion, chopped.

2 cloves garlic, minced.

1 large, sweet potato peeled and cubed.

1 cup red lentils, rinsed.

5 cups vegetable broth

1 teaspoon turmeric

1 teaspoon cumin

Salt and pepper to taste

Fresh cilantro for garnish

Instructions:

Heat olive oil in a large pot over moderate heat.

Add onion and garlic, and sauté until translucent.

Add sweet potato, red lentils, vegetable broth, turmeric, and cumin. Season with salt and pepper.

Bring to a boil, then reduce heat and simmer until sweet potatoes and lentils are tender, about 20 minutes.

Blend the soup until smooth, if desired. Garnish with fresh cilantro before serving.

Zucchini Basil Soup

Ingredients:

2 tablespoons olive oil
1 onion, chopped.
2 cloves garlic, minced.
4 cups chopped zucchini.
4 cups vegetable broth
1/2 cup fresh basil leaves, plus more for garnish
Salt and pepper to taste
Lemon juice (from 1 lemon)

Instructions:

In a large pot, heat olive oil over medium heat.

Add onion and garlic, sautéing until the onion is translucent.

Add the chopped zucchini and cook for about 5 minutes, until slightly softened.

Pour in the vegetable broth and bring the mixture to a simmer. Let it cook until the zucchini is very tender, about 15 minutes.

Add the fresh basil leaves and use an immersion blender to puree the soup until smooth.

Season with salt, pepper, and lemon juice to taste.

Blend again briefly to mix.

Serve the soup hot, garnished with additional basil leaves.

Tomato and White Bean Soup

Ingredients:

2 tablespoons olive oil

1 onion, diced.

2 cloves garlic, minced.

1 can (14 oz) diced tomatoes, with their juice.

1 can (14 oz) white beans drained and rinsed.

4 cups vegetable broth

1 teaspoon dried oregano

1 teaspoon dried basil

Salt and pepper to taste

Fresh parsley, chopped for garnish.

Instructions:

Heat olive oil in a large pot over medium heat.

Add the onion and garlic, cooking until the onion is soft and translucent.

Stir in the diced tomatoes (with juice), white beans, vegetable broth, oregano, and basil.

Season with salt and pepper.

Bring the soup to a boil, then reduce the heat and let it simmer for about 20 minutes to blend the flavors.

Use an immersion blender to partially puree the soup if a thicker consistency is desired, leaving some beans and tomatoes whole for texture.

Adjust the seasoning as needed and serve hot, garnished with fresh parsley.

Spinach and Green Pea Soup

Ingredients:

2 tablespoons olive oil

1 onion, chopped.

2 cloves garlic, minced.

4 cups vegetable broth

3 cups fresh spinach leaves

1 cup frozen green peas

Salt and pepper to taste

Mint leaves for garnish (optional)

A squeeze of lemon juice (optional)

Instructions:

In a large pot, heat olive oil over medium heat.

Add the onion and garlic, cooking until the onion is soft.

Add the vegetable broth to the pot and bring to a simmer.

Stir in the spinach leaves and green peas.

Continue to cook until the spinach has wilted, and the peas are tender, about 5 minutes.

Use an immersion blender to puree the soup until smooth.

Season with salt and pepper to taste. For a tangy flavor, add a squeeze of lemon juice.

Serve the soup hot, garnished with mint leaves for a fresh touch.

SNACKS

RECIPE

SNACKS RECIPE
Avocado and Tomato Salsa on Cucumber Slices

Ingredients:

1 ripe avocado, diced.

1 small tomato, diced.

1/4 red onion finely chopped.

Juice of 1 lime

Salt and pepper to taste

1 cucumber, sliced into rounds.

Instructions:

In a bowl, mix the diced avocado, tomato, and red onion.

Add lime juice, salt, and pepper, and gently toss to combine.

Place a spoonful of the mixture on each cucumber slice and serve.

Roasted Chickpeas

Ingredients:

1 can (15 oz) chickpeas drained and rinsed.

1 tablespoon olive oil

1/2 teaspoon smoked paprika.

1/2 teaspoon garlic powder

Salt to taste

Instructions:

Preheat your oven to 400°F (200°C).

Dry the chickpeas with a kitchen towel, removing any skins that come off.

Toss the chickpeas with olive oil, smoked paprika, garlic powder, and salt.

Spread on a baking sheet and roast for 20-30 minutes until crispy.

Let them cool before snacking.

Vegan Cheese and Apple Slices

Ingredients:

1 apple cored and sliced.

Vegan cheese, sliced.

Instructions:

Simply place a slice of vegan cheese on each apple slice and enjoy.

Zucchini Chips

Ingredients:

1 zucchini thinly sliced.

1 tablespoon olive oil

Salt and pepper to taste

Instructions:

Preheat your oven to 225°F (105°C).

Toss zucchini slices with olive oil, salt, and pepper.

Place on a baking sheet lined with parchment paper and bake for 1-2 hours, flipping halfway through, until crisp.

Almond Butter Stuffed Dates

Ingredients:

Medjool dates, pitted.

Almond butter

Instructions:

Open the dates slightly and fill each one with almond butter.

Serve as a sweet, nutrient-rich treat.

Veggie Sticks with Hummus

Ingredients:

Carrot sticks

Celery sticks

Bell pepper slices

1 cup hummus

Instructions:

Simply serve the veggie sticks with hummus for dipping.

Spiced Pumpkin Seeds

Ingredients:

1 cup pumpkin seeds cleaned and dried.

1 tablespoon olive oil

1/2 teaspoon cumin

1/2 teaspoon chili powder

Salt to taste

Instructions:

Preheat your oven to 300°F (150°C).

Toss pumpkin seeds with olive oil, cumin, chili powder, and salt.

Bake for about 45 minutes, stirring occasionally, until golden and crunchy.

Baked Kale Chips

Ingredients:

1 bunch kale, stems removed, and leaves torn.

1 tablespoon olive oil

Salt to taste

Instructions:

Preheat your oven to 300°F (150°C).

Toss kale leaves with olive oil and salt.

Bake for 20-25 minutes, until crisp, turning halfway through.

Edamame with Sea Salt

Ingredients:

1 cup frozen edamame, in pods

Sea salt to taste

Instructions:

Boil the edamame in water for 5-6 minutes, or microwave according to package instructions.

Drain and sprinkle with sea salt. Serve warmly.

Coconut Yogurt and Berry Parfait

Ingredients:

Coconut yogurt

Mixed berries (strawberries, blueberries, raspberries)

A sprinkle of chia seeds

Instructions:

In a glass, layer coconut yogurt and mixed berries.

Top with a sprinkle of chia seeds for added nutrition.

CONCLUSION

In " Plant Based Insulin Resistance Diet For PCOS" We have embarked on a transformative journey, exploring how a carefully curated vegan diet can significantly impact those managing PCOS and insulin resistance. Through the comprehensive guide provided, including detailed recipes for breakfast, lunch, dinner, soups, and snacks, we have seen that adopting a plant-based diet does not mean compromising on variety, taste, or nutrition. Instead, it opens a world of vibrant, healthful eating options that can help stabilize blood sugar levels, support hormonal balance, and promote overall well-being.

Living with PCOS and insulin resistance requires a holistic approach to health, and diet plays a crucial role in this process. The vegan diet, rich in fruits, vegetables, legumes, nuts, and seeds, provides a powerful tool for combating the challenges associated with these conditions. It's not just about managing symptoms; it's about thriving despite them.

As you incorporate these recipes and dietary strategies into your life, remember that change doesn't happen overnight. It's about making consistent, mindful choices that contribute to your health and happiness. Listen to your body, be patient with yourself, and don't hesitate to seek support from healthcare professionals, nutritionists, and the PCOS community.

This book is not just a collection of recipes; it's a testament to the strength and resilience of those managing PCOS and insulin resistance every day. It's a reminder that with the right resources and support, you can take control of your health and lead a vibrant, fulfilling life. Whether you're newly diagnosed or have been navigating this path for some time, let this book be a companion on your journey to wellness, one meal at a time.

DAILY
MEAL PLANNER

BREAKFAST

LUNCH

DINNER

SHOPPING LIST

DAILY MEAL PLANNER

BREAKFAST

LUNCH

DINNER

SHOPPING LIST

DAILY
MEAL PLANNER

BREAKFAST

LUNCH

DINNER

SHOPPING LIST

DAILY MEAL PLANNER

BREAKFAST

LUNCH

DINNER

SHOPPING LIST

DAILY MEAL PLANNER

BREAKFAST

LUNCH

DINNER

SHOPPING LIST

DAILY
MEAL PLANNER

BREAKFAST

LUNCH

DINNER

SHOPPING LIST

DAILY MEAL PLANNER

BREAKFAST

LUNCH

DINNER

SHOPPING LIST

DAILY MEAL PLANNER

BREAKFAST

LUNCH

DINNER

SHOPPING LIST

DAILY
MEAL PLANNER

BREAKFAST

LUNCH

DINNER

SHOPPING LIST

DAILY MEAL PLANNER

BREAKFAST

LUNCH

DINNER

SHOPPING LIST

DAILY MEAL PLANNER

BREAKFAST

LUNCH

DINNER

SHOPPING LIST

DAILY MEAL PLANNER

BREAKFAST

LUNCH

DINNER

SHOPPING LIST

DAILY MEAL PLANNER

BREAKFAST

LUNCH

DINNER

SHOPPING LIST

DAILY MEAL PLANNER

BREAKFAST

LUNCH

DINNER

SHOPPING LIST

DAILY
MEAL PLANNER

BREAKFAST

LUNCH

DINNER

SHOPPING LIST

DAILY
MEAL PLANNER

BREAKFAST

LUNCH

DINNER

SHOPPING LIST

DAILY MEAL PLANNER

BREAKFAST

LUNCH

DINNER

SHOPPING LIST

DAILY
MEAL PLANNER

BREAKFAST

LUNCH

DINNER

SHOPPING LIST

DAILY
MEAL PLANNER

BREAKFAST

LUNCH

DINNER

SHOPPING LIST

DAILY MEAL PLANNER

BREAKFAST

LUNCH

DINNER

SHOPPING LIST

DAILY
MEAL PLANNER

BREAKFAST

LUNCH

DINNER

SHOPPING LIST

DAILY MEAL PLANNER

BREAKFAST

LUNCH

DINNER

SHOPPING LIST

DAILY
MEAL PLANNER

BREAKFAST

LUNCH

DINNER

SHOPPING LIST

DAILY
MEAL PLANNER

BREAKFAST

LUNCH

DINNER

SHOPPING LIST

DAILY
MEAL PLANNER

BREAKFAST

LUNCH

DINNER

SHOPPING LIST

DAILY
MEAL PLANNER

BREAKFAST

LUNCH

DINNER

SHOPPING LIST

DAILY MEAL PLANNER

BREAKFAST

LUNCH

DINNER

SHOPPING LIST

DAILY MEAL PLANNER

BREAKFAST

LUNCH

DINNER

SHOPPING LIST

DAILY MEAL PLANNER

BREAKFAST

LUNCH

DINNER

SHOPPING LIST

DAILY MEAL PLANNER

BREAKFAST

LUNCH

DINNER

SHOPPING LIST